RELENT LESS WEIGHT LOSS

How To Easily And Relentlessly Lose Weight throughout the year Without Gaining it Back

Dr. Chio Ugochukwu

Copyright © 2018 Dr. Chio Ugochukwu

All Rights Reserved. No part of this book may be reproduced in any form, or means, without the permission of the author or publisher.

Published by Bundant Enterprises

3053 Rancho Vista Blvd, H-197

Palmdale, California

ISBN-13:978-1720456179

ISBN-10:1720456178

Printed in the United States of America.

Disclaimer and Terms of Use

The author and publisher have made every effort to ensure the accuracy and completeness of the information contained in this book, we assume no responsibility for errors or omissions therein. It is solely for informational and educational purposes and should not be regarded as a substitute for professional advice. Your reliance upon information and content obtained through this book is solely at your own risk. The author and publisher assume no liability or responsibility for any adverse consequences for the use of any product, information, idea or instruction contained in this book.

Dedication

This book is dedicated to all those who want to easily and relentlessly lose weight throughout the year without gaining it back.

Acknowledgement

I want to acknowledge the tremendous support I have received from my family, friends and those who inspire me by their refusal to quit.

Table of Contents

"THE ABILITY

TO TAKE FOCUSED ACTION EVERYDAY

TOWARDS YOUR DAILY GOAL

IS THE DIFFERENCE BETWEEN LIVING

THE LIFESTYLE OF YOUR DREAMS AND

DREAMING OF YOUR LIFESTYLE"

DR. CHIO

Introduction

Did you know that more people die from eating too much than from not having enough to eat? Did you know that according to the World Health Organization (WHO), the number of obese people in the world has almost tripled since 1975? The total number of overweight adults in 2016 was almost 2 billion, with over 650 million obese (WHO, 2017). According to the WHO, body mass index (BMI) above 25 is overweight and BMI 30 and above is obese.

Did you know that if you are overweight or obese that you are at an increased risk of having diseases like diabetes, hypertension, and heart disease? Did you know that about 300,000 people die every year from obesity-related health problems in the United States (Samaranayake, Ong, Leung,& Chueng,

2012)? Did you know that most people who are overweight as children struggle with weight – related problems as adults?

Did you know that despite the fact that the factors that lead to obesity are well known, the unhealthy habits that lead to its occurrence such as poor nutrition, lack of exercise and poor lifestyle choices are difficulty to change (Anshel, 2010)? Why? The reason is that people give up they get permanent results. They are not relentless. They begin weight loss programs with enthusiasm but they get derailed by circumstance, inconsistency, social conditions and lack of focus.

If you truly want to lose weight and keep it off, you have to be clear on why you want to lose weight and how you will do it. While you may want to lose weight because you want your clothes to fit better, get in shape, have more fun or look younger, don't forget your health. Remember that in the United States and worldwide, obesity is associated with some of the leading causes of death like hypertension, heart disease and respiratory disease (CDC, WHO, 2017).

How will you lose weight? What steps, actions or activities will you do everyday to help you lose weight? Through this book you will learn how the relentless weight loss program will help you lose weight and keep it off throughout the year. To consistently lose weight, you have to stay focused and centered in the moment and ignore the daily distractions, criticisms and annoyances that are invariably part of your daily life.

Ask yourself what you have done in the last 24 hours to help you lose weight and keep it off. Did you keep to your personalized weight loss plan? Have you developed your own personalized weight loss plan? Unless you consistently take the actions that will help you fulfill your goals, even after you have discovered why you want to lose weight, you would find yourself losing and gaining weight every week!

One of the secrets to fearlessly losing weight is the ability to let disappointments or unmet expectations go and continue to take consistent daily action towards your goal of relentless weight loss. Don't dwell on your disappointments or goals that you failed to meet. Learn from them and move on.

No matter where are you are in your weight loss journey, **Relentless Weight loss**, which is based on the compass method, will help reach your goals faster. The compass method is a holistic system for relentless transformation that is based on the 7 compass profiles. It is the core method that I will use in the pathways or steps for relentless weight loss that I will share with you in this book. How much weight do you want to lose? How much weight can you successfully lose everyday will depend on the actions you take every hour of the day. Do you want to easily and relentlessly lose weight and keep it off?

TIPS FOR THE DAY

BE PREPARED TO LOSE WEIGHT

DESPITE

DAILY

SETBACKS OR CHALLENGES

ONCE YOU START YOUR WEIGHT LOSS

JOURNEY

YOU

HAVE

TO

PERSIST UNTIL SUCCESS HAPPENS

(PUSH)

Make your weight loss holistic

Did you know that everything you do affects your weight? Do you have an everything-related or holistic approach to weight loss? Don't assume that because you failed in your previous attempts at losing weight that you will fail again. Invest in yourself. Make your weight loss holistic! Do you know how the different aspects of the compass profile can help you do better?

Did you know that you can relentlessly pursue your daily goals through the use of the compass profiles? The compass health profiles are the foundation for the compass method for transformational living. The components of the compass profile are:

C = Community Relationships profile.

O = Operational capacity profile.

M= Metabolic profile.

P= Physical profile.

A= Ambition profile.

S= Spiritual profile.

S = Self Knowledge profile.

How can you use these profiles to lose weight throughout the year? **The community relationships profile is essentially your communications profile.** The first step in using the community relationships profile is to gain a deeper understanding of yourself and others. Communicate with yourself first and write down your deepest fears and worries. What is affecting your confidence in yourself and your ability to make decisions? What is holding you back from making a commitment to relentless weight loss? Is it fear of the process or fear of communication with others?

Effective communication is good because it will help you to reduce stress. The more you reduce stress the less likely you will attempt to use eating to keep stress off. Do the best you can and leave the rest. **The smallest action is better than the greatest intention.** Taking action will help you reduce stress and have more energy for all the fun things you would like to do with your life. Try to reduce complex problems to small segments that you can accomplish. Begin where you are, not where you want to be.

Ask yourself questions that will help you recognize which aspects of your relationship with others could either be contributing to your weight gain or making it more difficult for you to lose weight. Remember that when you are communicating with others, they will interact with you from their own perspective, worldview, personality or experience. Their own personal interest will drive the relationship more than equity or the truth. Don't let this frustrate you or disrupt your focus on losing weight. Keep in mind that everything affects your weight loss and narrow your focus to finding out more about how you can consistently implement your daily strategy for weight loss.

What is your operational capacity profile? Your operational capacity is your ability to get things done or to make adjustments when they are required. What is your wherewithal for achieving your goals? If you don't have the money to fly to New York, do you consider other ways to get there like driving, taking a bus or train or do you simply give up? What is your operational capacity for weight loss? Do you have a process and strategy in place that fits your worldview and personality that will help you lose weight? Through your **operational capacity profile,** you will learn how to analyze things for yourself, how to get things done and how you can continue to achieve your goals by improving daily. A weight loss journal will help you keep track of the different aspects of your weight loss journey.

You have to think of weight loss from January to December, not just in January after the holidays. Remember that it is easier to prevent yourself from gaining weight than to lose weight after you have gained it. This is why the focus of the relentless weight loss program is year round. The holiday season from November to December, is full of festivities and celebrations in which you are continually asked to eat more and more.

If you want to lose weight all year round, you have a holistic approach that includes all the circumstances and situations that make up your day. If you are not sure of the operational capacity that will work best for you, look back at your life and find out which method of preparation and execution has worked the best for you in your most successful projects. Modify your weight loss strategy to fit that model.

Include in your project review, things like getting ready for vacations, birthday parties or getting ready for a wedding or tasks as simple as going to work on time and cleaning your house. For most people, the best way to tackle most projects is to start on time and break them down into small simple steps. For others every project is eventually done at the last minute. You cannot lose weight and keep it off through last minute approaches.

If you like to get things done at the last minute, it means you tend to procrastinate and underestimate how much time you would need to get your projects completed. **You have to learn to persist and win strategically (PAWS). Remember that inadequate preparation leads to failure.** To lose weight and keep it off, you have to start with a small plan and build on it slowly, in a way that suits your internal and external circumstances. You have to use your PAWS to get your target.

Do you know your metabolic profile? When was the last time you did your blood work done? Your **metabolic profile** will include both your nutritional and metabolic analysis. You can get your metabolic analysis by getting your physiological and laboratory tests done. This will help you to know if there are significant medical problems responsible for your weight struggles. Getting the right tests done with the help of a healthcare professional or your doctor will make it easy for you to know which aspect of your health profile you need to focus on improving.

When it comes to losing weight even without running tests, **your family history can help**

you a get a better picture of your risk factors. If you have a family history of diabetes, hypertension, kidney disease or chronic obesity, then you have to be much more vigilant than others.

The best way to analyze the nutritional component of your compass metabolic profile is to do your 72- hour food audit. You can do this with your food journal or with your diary.

The Physical Profile includes your weight, height, waist circumference and BMI (Body Mass Index). It also includes your heart rate and lung function. These factors are important because it is important to know your health status before you can engage in vigorous exercise. **Take action today, weigh yourself today, even if you feel you are in excellent health.**

Exercise everyday. Keep it simple. Do daily mild to moderate activities like **walking**, dancing, jump ropes and pushups. If you are more interested in vigorous exercise like going to the gym for intense workouts or playing basketball, tennis, and baseball, you need to remember to check with your doctor to make sure that you are healthy enough to begin vigorous exercise.

One advantage of staying physically active is that it helps you burn off excessive calories that would have been converted to fat. Increased storage of excess energy in the form of fat will ultimately build up your weight and cause more health problems. In the relentless weight program you have to exercise everyday!

What is your ambition profile? **The Ambition Profile** assesses your drive and motivation.

What is the highest level of success you would strive for in your endeavors? Would like to lose weight and keep it off permanently or would like to lose weight for an event or an occasion only? You can use the ambition profile to **set measurable goals like losing your first 10 pounds within the first 3 months of starting the *relentless weight loss* program.**

This is an important strategy because once you can confidently write down the actions and activities that helped you lose your first 10 pounds, you can build on it to lose more pounds. What is your ambition profile? Write it down as part of relentless weight program.

The remaining two profiles are **Spirituality and Self Knowledge**, both of which examine your psychosocial and spiritual make up. They will help you have a **better understanding of your personality,** character and connection with God and the universe. **Knowing your personality type will give you a greater insight into how your sense of self affects your weight loss strategy.**

A better understanding of your psychosocial strengths and weaknesses will help you know your limitations, when it comes to choosing pathways to better health and consistent weight loss. It will also help you to anticipate problems, challenges and pressure points.

On the spiritual side of the equation, more and more studies are beginning to show that those who meditate or are truly prayerful are better able to handle health challenges than those who do neither. Of course I realize that there are different interpretations of what it means to be spiritual and that one size does not fit all.

Through the use of the 7 elements of the compass profile you will be able develop a more holistic approach to your weight loss. The next step in your *relentless weight loss* is doing your 72 –hour food audit.

TIPS FOR THE DAY

DON'T LET THE PERFECT BECOME THE ENEMY OF THE POSSIBLE

WRITE DOWN A SENTENCE THAT BEST EXPLAINS YOUR HOLISTIC UNDERSTANDING OF YOURSELF.

KNOW YOUR STRENGTHS, WEAKNESSES, AND WORLDVIEW

Do your 72 -hour food audit and self-analysis

What did you have for breakfast 3 days ago? Was it healthy? Did you snack on fruits or on chips? Do you the patterns that dominate your relationships, activities and eating habits? Use the first 24 hours or first day of your food audit to learn as much as you can about yourself. Write down the patterns that are most prominent in your life during the past 72 hours in your weight loss journal. Identify and write down your:

*Eating pattern

*Working pattern

*Relationship pattern

*Activity pattern

*And Meditation pattern.

Write down your meals and snacks, how much TV you watch, and how you typically deal with your emotions like anger and sadness. Be accurate and specific.

In the second 24 hours or second day set up an appointment with your health care provider to get a more detailed picture of your metabolic profile, especially your cholesterol level and other tests relevant to your family and medical history. Do you have a family or personal history of obesity – related illnesses like diabetes, high blood pressure, heart attack or stroke? Consider taking advantage of free informational health exams or blood work offered at your office or your membership clubs or insurance to get your cholesterol or metabolic profile. If you are not able to do this, work with results from your first 24 hours of assessment.

In the third 24 hours or third day which will complete your 72 hour time frame begin to write down the components of your healthy living blueprint for the Long haul. Make this your own personalized list of actions and pledges that will help you transform your health and life. This basically means taking some detailed transformative actions and applying them to yourself and your circumstances.

Here is an example of a list you can make on the third day of your 72 hour time frame:

*If you smoke, quit smoking now or plan to stop.

*Eat more grains, vegetables, fruits, milk and beans, and use oils like cranola and olive oils.

*Eat at least 10 grams of fibers daily through eating nuts and cereals like oats

*** Stop eating processed food like bread and pizza.**

*Eat at least five servings of fruits and vegetables daily.

*Eat a delicious red apple with every meal.

*Read your nutritional facts before you buy or use your food products.

*Cut down your food portions by at least one-third.

*Eat your food in one location without TV or your smart phone.

*Eat fish and skinless poultry like chicken or turkey.

*Drink low-fat milk or eat low fat yoghurt.

*Walk at least 45 minutes everyday.

*Keep stress out of your relationships.

*Sleep at least six to eight hours a day.

*Cut down on unnecessary expenses.

*Call a friend today.

*Review your finances.

*Help at least one person each day.

*Meditate or say a prayer or do both.

*Form a healthy living-group of friends and family members.

*Write down your feelings and experiences.

*Repeat your blood pressure check.

*Weigh yourself every 3 days.

*Take Omega 3, vitamin D, Magnesium, lutein and vitamin C everyday..

*Keep your appointment with your healthcare providers.

*Keep eating right even after a lapse.

*Do your yearly physical.

*Do your screening tests as recommended by your healthcare providers.

*Become familiar with your family and medical history.

*Review your health insurance regularly.

*Get more education.

*Protect your home from falls and accidents.

*Work for the future everyday.

*Continue to write down your emotions periodically.

*Forgive yourself and others daily.

*Keep quiet if you have nothing positive to say.

*Review and modify this list as it fits your individual needs and circumstances.

There you have it! These are the elements of the individualized 72 hour blueprint for **relentless weight loss.** You are welcome to use them and begin to lose weight everyday for the rest of the year! Instead floating a weight loss trial balloon, read the next chapter for more ideas and thoughts on how you can develop specific, realistic and achievable goals for relentless weight loss.

.

TIPS FOR THE DAY

STAY STRONG

REMEMBER THAT SUCCESS DEPENDS ON CONSISTENCY AND PERSISTENCE

Set specific achievable weight loss goals with realistic strategies

When will you achieve your weight loss goals? Have you set the specific actions you will take everyday to help you lose weight? If you really want lose weight and keep it off, you have to set goals you can achieve with realistic strategies. Don't set a goal of losing 100 pounds in 1 week by going to the gym 24 hours a day for 1 week. It is neither realistic nor achievable. This is particularly the case if you have to go to work everyday and still take care of your family. **Unachievable goals lead to discouragement.**

Making your goals achievable and realistic combines the compass operational capacity profile "O" and the ambition profile "A" in the compass method. The good news is that **when you set an**

achievable goal like losing weight and keeping it off, your focus will narrow and you will waste less time with the resources at hand. Life will support you in every possible way and provide what you need to make fearless progress in your journey.

Don't let your daily struggles, distractions, frustrations and criticisms prevent you from striving to live up to your full potential. You have the potential to do anything you want to do including relentlessly losing weight throughout the year. **Believe in yourself!** You have all the resources you require and enough skills to live the life you intended. You can do this by believing in yourself and taking action and staying focused on achieving your daily goals one step at a time. Have you set specific hourly weight loss goals to get you through the day? If you haven't, do it not later than today.

What are your specific weight loss goals for the day? What will you do when you feel the urge to eat ice cream? What will you do when your friends urge you to try a sugar-loaded salty delight? If you truly want to relentlessly lose weight, you have to learn to have a specific optimistic focus for the hours that make up your day. If you do not do this, you will not have an anchor to help you stay committed to effective implementation. Instead you will end up not finishing the mini-projects that will help you accomplish your weekly weight loss goals.

In order to lose weight relentlessly, you have to consistently remind yourself to take productive action and stop allowing distractions like negative thinking and purposeless action take away your focus and keep you from achieving your daily weight-loss goals. Say "No", to the urge to eat ice cream, to try a salty delight or to simply eat more cake. Eat them when they fit into your plans and not simply because others will feel bad or think you are different because you refused.

When you have realistic strategies for weight loss, taking specific steps to accomplish your goals become easier. This will help you to focus on what you can do to make things positive rather than worrying about failures and outcomes when setbacks or unexpected events happen in your life. It is being part of the solution rather than the cause. **Taking action on your positive thoughts is essential to relentless weight loss.**

Your potential is unlimited and you can achieve anything you set your mind to. As you strive to fearlessly lose weight, you will discover that there will be additional distractions and challenges. You have to be aware of the different distractions and attractions that occur throughout the year. Birthday parties, graduation ceremonies, weddings, holidays and anniversaries occur throughout the year and may disrupt your well-crafted weight loss plans unless you take proactive action. Do you have a plan for celebrations? Do you snack with fruits before parties so that you won't overeat and blow up weight loss plan at the party? Do you watch what you drink? Do you reassess your focus every 15 minutes? Are you wasting time or are accomplishing your set mini-goals for the day? The relentless weight loss program requires consistent vigilance and action. Stay focused.

This may sometimes be more challenging than you would expect because your mind may remind of your previous struggles and failures with weight loss. What will you do? You can use the compass "VAM" method to make changes to your daily meals and eating habit so that you can easily achieve your specific and realistic weight loss goals.

TIPS FOR THE DAY

SET YOUR DAILY EXERCISE GOALS.

USE THE COMPASS "VAM" METHOD OF VARIETY, ADJUSTMENT AND MODERATION TO CONTROL YOUR DAILY EATING HABITS

ADD MORE VEGGIES TO YOUR MEAL EVERY DAY.

REDUCE YOUR FOOD PORTIONS

CUT OUT PROCESSED FOOD

WEIGHT YOURSELF EVERY WEEK.

SAY "NO" MORE OFTEN.

Use the compass "VAM" method to manage your daily meals and lose weight relentlessly

Do you have the discipline to do easy activities daily? Did you know that you can lose weight throughout the year by sticking to a simple strategy everyday? Do you know how you can Use the compass "VAM" method to achieve your specific weight loss goals?

You can easily build up your confidence in your ability to consistently lose weight through **the compass "VAM" method for relentless weight loss** that is based on **variety, adjustments and moderation.** The order in which you make the modifications is entirely up to you.

A suggested first strategy would be for you to start by reducing the food portion of your daily meals.

The first step towards implementing your compass "VAM" method for relentless weight loss is to cut down the servings or portions of your regular meal by half. This will reduce your energy intake by about half or a third. You fill the gap with vegetables and fruits. If you feel pangs of hunger, snack with nuts, drink plenty of water or eat some fruits.

Why is the reduction in portions so important? According to surveys by doctors and nutritionists the average American male takes about 3,000 calories per day and the female 2,400 calories per day (Reuters Health, 2015). According to Dr. Wang an energy intake and expenditure expert, consistent loss or reduction in energy intake of 100 calories would lead to 10 pounds loss in weight (Reuters Health, 2015). **This means that without knowing the exact quantity of calories you eat, you can continue to reduce your meal, snack or**

social eating portions until you notice your first loss of 10 pounds and use it for a marker or foundation for all your future weight-loss strategies.

The more you reduce your servings, the more weight you would lose because the fewer calories you will take in, the less excess calories you will have to store as fat. However, reduced servings may mean more hunger pangs. This is a serious potential problem that could make you drink a lot of soda or eat many hot dogs as an immediate way of dealing with your hunger pangs. Unless you make adjustments this could simply lead you to more energy intake and more weight gain.

The next step in the compass "VAM" method is to make adjustments. Adjustments are changes you make to eating pattern and your meals so that you can continue to lose weight and keep it off.

Drinking more soda is the wrong **adjustment** for hunger pangs from portion reduction. The right **adjustment** would be to eat more fruits, vegetables and fibers as fillers. Fibers are especially good for your system because they help to increase bowel movement. This has the added effect of making your digestive system more efficient.

Sometimes the adjustment you can make will be affected by your culture. For different cultures and settings, different modifications to familiar eating habits can be made. In the United States this would entail cutting down on fast foods, soda and other processed foods. According to the CDC sugar-sweetened beverages (SSBs) or sugary drinks like sodas are leading sources of added sugars in the American diet. Drinking soda is associated with weight gain/obesity, type 2 diabetes, gout, tooth decay, heart disease, kidney diseases, and liver disease (CDC, 2017). If you want to lose weight throughout the year you have to stop drinking sugar-sweetened beverages like soda, fruit-juice and fruit punch. **Drink water or unsweetened tea instead of soda.**

Do not go along with food choices that will not be good for your health just because people from your culture may challenge you or make fun of you. Your culture is supposed to help you, not to kill you. You can do this by finding a way to eat right within your culture. If you cannot completely eliminate fast food cut it down to once a month.

Another adjustment could be to stop eating processed food like bread. Did you know that bread can be a source of sodium and too much energy intake? Did you know that on the average a slide of bread contains 150 mg of sodium and 110 calories per serving? This would mean that for bread with one slice per serving, 10 slices would be 1100calories. This would be more than half of the average 2000 calories per day recommended for most people.

Do you know why you have gained weight though you're exercising more? If you are eating in moderation by cutting down your portions, eating fruits and vegetables and doing regular exercise but have not lost weight, you wonder why. The first reason may be because you have not cut down on the daily amount of sugar you eat every day. Though the recommended daily sugar intake for men is about 36 g or 9 teaspoons and 25 g or 6 teaspoons for women, Americans eat about 3 times this value everyday (AHA). This is because most people end up eating varieties of candy and drinking soda everyday. Did you know that in past 30 years more and more sugar has been added the American diet (AHA)? The more sugar you eat the more calories you shall eat that will make you continue gain weight despite the reduction in portion size and increase in exercise.

The second reason may be related to your snacking habits. Did you know that one small pack of unsalted pea nuts contained 220 calories per serving but 6 servings per pack? How does this information which you read from the nutrition facts on the pack help you? It can help you determine calories per pack, sodium per pack and sugar per pack

.

Be careful with snacks!!! Did you know that when you finish a pack of pea nuts rich in dietary fiber, with little or zero sodium and cholesterol, you are also eating more than more 1000 calories. When you combine it with 1100 calories from 10 slices of bread, it means that from bread and peanuts alone, give you have more than 2000 calories already eaten (1100+1320=2420) calories. This shows that though you had reduced your calories per meal through reducing your portion per meal, because you had not paid careful attention to size or frequency of your snacks, you were still eating a lot of calories per day through snacks.

If you want to lose weight and keep it off, you have to know your daily sources of extra calories. Do you know how many calories you have in your morning cereal or pack of pea nuts? When you regularly read the nutritional facts in the food you eat, you can find out calories per serving. When you know the calories per serving you can more realistically adjust your portion size to cut down on your daily calories intake

If you are eating a lot of nuts, check your nutrition facts as soon as possible. When I checked mine I discovered that I was eating more calories through my snacks than I expected. I cut my snack portions by more than half. This helped me reduce my extra calories by more than half. This adjustment helped me to start losing weight more consistently and keeping it off. You can do the same after a full examination of your own snacking habits.

You do not have to do a full detailed calories count to know your average energy intake. You can get a good idea of your calories intake by doing your own 72-hour food audit. This will help you identify the highest and most frequent source of calories in your daily meals. All you have to do is to remember that you have to reduce all sources of your daily intake of calories from your meals to your snacks. Do this to a level that allows you to feel full, eat healthy and still lose weight. Remember that it is calories in, calories out!

Apart from the adjustments I have mentioned so far, another easy one, you can quickly do, is to start drinking a glass of water before each meal. This will make feel full, without eating as much as before. After a while, you will be able to consistently cut down on your daily portions of food or snacks.

Research has shown that drinking water before a meal will help to expand your stomach. This approach will make you feel completely full when you are only 80% full. This is important because eating only up to 80 % full was one of the common practices of people of Okinawa in Japan, who have the highest number of centenarians in the world (Boyle & Long, 2010). If you want to lose relentlessly without making it seem like a tedious task then drink at least two glasses of water per meal and increase the bulk in your meals through fruits and vegetables. **This will help you reduce**

your total calorie intake per meal without tortures diets.

To increase your intake of fruits and vegetables, start by eating every meal with salads consisting of cabbage, tomatoes, carrots, broccoli, spinach and bananas. Eating a colorful variety of fruits and vegetables per meal with reduced portions of brown rice will make your meal significantly more healthy and more bulky but less energy dense. It will help you to lose significant pounds and keep them off. **Remember calories in calories out.**

You need to be careful when you start cutting down on calories by reducing the intake of carbohydrate like white bread, white rice or pasta. This will make you lose weight quickly because it is usually stored in the body as glycogen which contains water. You need to be careful because the brain gets most of its energy from glucose and if it does not get enough you begin to feel tired, weak, unable to sleep and ill. Unless you switch to fiber-rich carbohydrate sources like baked sweet potato, whole grain bread, barley, oat meal and brown rice, you may end up quitting after a few weeks. This is why **the Compass "VAM" Method is based on variety, adjustments and moderation (VAM).**

To make sustainable adjustments and modifications to your meals concentrate on variety and moderation. Include chicken, fish, beans, cottage cheese, chia seeds or low fat yogurt in your meals. You can make low fat yogurt and chia seed your breakfast.Have eggs, nuts and red meat occasionally. You can further reduce your fat intake by eating skinless chicken or turkey. Turkey and chicken have their fat on their skin but red meat has most of its fat contained within the meat. Grilling is better than frying, and always aim to use unsaturated oils like corn, and olive oils for cooking.

You can also gradually reduce the fat content in your milk products. You can do this by changing the variety of milk that you drink from whole milk, to 2% fat; then to 1% fat. I am wary of fat free milk because it is still important to get fat in your body which can be used through cellular metabolism to produce cell membranes and hormones. Choose lower-fat cheese and yogurt. When you buy yogurt, also check that it does not contain sugar. The good thing about reducing to 1% fat milk is that it remains tasteful. Fat has 9 calories of energy per gram compared to carbohydrate and proteins that have about 4 per gram.

Remember that variety is the spice of life. It is the "V" in the compass "VAM" method. Do not eat the same meal day in day out. Why? It gets boring after a while and you will soon find yourself looking less excited about eating healthy. You have to like and enjoy what you eat. **Weight loss is not punishment!**

To sustainably lose weight, you have to aim for a healthy variety of food that contains adequate but moderate portions of fat, proteins, carbohydrates and vitamins. Eat enough food to fill full, when you eat. If you don't feel full after a meal you will find yourself eating too much sugary snacks in between meals to make you feel full. This will make you gain back weight you may have lost. If you feel hungry between meals, snack with small portions of almonds, cashew nuts or peanuts. Almonds will make you feel less hungry and still boost your metabolism, though they take getting used. Have you tried almonds before? Please share your thoughts in the compass club.

Make variety part of your daily eating habit. Do not eat a particular food too much just because you like it. If usually eat to a lot of white bread and soda just because you enjoyed them, cut down your portions then consider stopping them altogether. This is because bread and soda contain significant calories and sodium. Strictly speaking, you have to watch how much soda or beer you drink. Beer has a lot of empty calories with little ingredients. Drinking too much beer may increase your belly fat without giving you adequate amounts of important vitamins like vitamin B 6. Another way to balance your meal would be to halve your intake of all pure or added fats as previously outlined.

If you plan your meals and snacks ahead of time you will have to make them the variety that will help you to relentlessly lose weight. Take time to plan at least one lunch and dinner every week without meat or cheese. Create your meals around whole grains, vegetables and beans to increase fiber and reduce fat. If you want to have something to chew on, get some fish or tofu. You can make every Friday your fish meal day to begin with then gradually add more and more fish to your meals.

Have at least five servings of fruit every day. Choose fruit that is in season. Take an apple per meal. The red delicious apples contain pectin, a fiber that helps to promote healthy cholesterol levels and contain more amounts of antioxidants than many other types of apples.

You now have a deeper understanding of yourself in terms of holistic weight loss, a specific and realistic weight loss goal and the compass "VAM" method to help you get the results you desire quickly. However, all the depth of knowledge and insight into losing weight and keep it off, will fail

unless you take action everyday!!!

TIPS FOR THE DAY

REDUCE YOUR FOOD PORTION BY HALF

VARIETY MATTERS: PUT MORE FRUITS AND VEGETABLES IN EACH MEAL

EAT MORE FISH AND WHOLE GRAINS

CUT DOWN ON RED MEAT

CUT DOWN ON SODA AND BEER

DRINK MORE WATER

EAT AN APPLE PER MEAL

PLAN YOUR SNACKS IN ADVANCE

CUT DOWN ON YOUR SNACK PORTIONS

TAKE ACTION EVERYDAY

READ YOUR NUTRITION FACTS

Take action everyday

Do you take action every day? Having achievable goals and realistic strategies will not help you lose weight unless you take action everyday. If you really want to relentlessly lose weight and fulfill your daily goals and live the lifestyle of your dreams, you have to stop assuming you will do things later. **Take action now! When you have a good idea, act on it immediately with whatever resources you have at hand.** Delaying taking action will lead to unintended consequences. Take action now instead of assuming you will act later.

Stop pointing fingers at others whenever things do not go as planned or you fail to do the things you should have done to help you lose weight.. After all, we all make mistakes. We all have room for improvement. If you focus on taking small but productive steps everyday, without allowing yourself to be bogged down by daily frustrations, challenges and criticisms you will gradually turn your life around and make it the amazing life you have always wanted it to be. Stop waiting for things to be perfect, act with what you have.

Take a deep breath and re-focus on the positive actions that can lead to the results you want. Look at the patterns or circumstances that usually lead to anxieties and troublesome behaviors that stop you from taking action everyday. Try as much as possible to modify these patterns everyday. This will help you avoid behavior that drains your energy and wastes your time. Time is a limited commodity so it has to be used wisely. **"Yesterday" used to be "Tomorrow".** Assuming you will do things later is one way of mismanaging time and making your gain weight daily instead of losing it.

Identify situations and events that make it difficult for you to get the results you want from your behavior. If everyone in your office is always urging you to eat food that you do not consider healthy, what will you do? Will you cave in? Will you refuse and or explain why you have to stick to your guns now? The more you can consistently take action everyday, the more you can consistently lose weight daily. Do not wait for the perfect preparation. Stop assuming you will start later because you may never start at all.

You cannot relentlessly lose weight daily and throughout the year if your days are dotted with unfinished or and uncompleted projects. Did you not know that not having a reliable and consistent approach to weight –loss can lead a pursuit of too many strategies with more anxiety, more stress and potentially more errors? Do you know that when you are distracted by lack of time, you end up rushing through your tasks without giving them the thorough attention they would require to produce great results?

This would include rushing through your food, your exercise routine and your communication strategies for dealing with unexpected challenges and setbacks. Trust the individualized process you have developed for yourself through the compass profiles and the compass "VAM" method for weight loss. Take action now!

When you begin to take daily action to lose weight, you will have successes and challenges. If you find yourself discouraged by what others might say or do, make an effort to communicate positively with yourself. If you don't, the negative comments and words of discouragement from others will challenge your ability to stay the course. Make your communication strategies part of your daily activities to help you lose weight and keep it off.

TIPS FOR THE DAY

TIME WAITS FOR NO ONE

GIVE YOUR BEST AND LEAVE THE REST

"YESTERDAY" USED TO BE "TOMORROW"

FOCUS

Use effective communication strategies to help yourself lose weight relentlessly

Do you know that communication is an important part of weight loss? Do you remember that the "C" in the compass method represents community relationships and communications? You can use your communication strategy to foresee and rule your daily encounters with others. If you are dealing with a difficult person or someone who is usually quick to judge or very negative in outlook be prepared to bend without breaking. Remember that most things in life are transitional, including such conversations. Don't let such negative conversations derail you from your goal of sustainable weight loss.

If you want to remain on track with your weight

loss program throughout your daily interactions everyday, you have to be able to recognize hidden antagonistic conversational messages and deal with them. Your inner voice can make a huge difference in your focus, success and ability to lose weight throughout the year.

After you have gained a deeper understanding of why you're bombarding yourself with negative thoughts you can use effective communication strategies to anticipate what you might say to yourself during certain situations and "rewrite" the dialogue. You can use effective communication strategies to encourage yourself to keep on trying to lose weight and keep it off, even when other factors like your job, social role, family dynamics and daily encounters with others push you in the opposite direction. If the dialogue doesn't quite go the way you planned it in your mind, you can do this through the EFRAMES communication strategy.

If you don't know about EFRAMES, read my book, "9 ways to keep stress out your relationships…" to get more details. In EFRAMES, "E" stands for "emphasizing empathy throughout your interactions with others". "F" stands for "find and focus on the facts", and "R" for read body language. "A" is for assessing relationship interactions. The remaining elements of the EFRAMES framework are "MES". M stands for maintain self-esteem in your interaction and relationships. "E" stands for evaluate everything in your interaction with others. **The elephant always looks different for everyone.** "S" stands for summarize your interactions through self–assertiveness while supporting your position with facts and being mindful of the other person's feelings.

When it comes to daily communications, it is important to pay particular attention to how you relate to your family, friends and.co-workers. Though your family may love you and genuinely want the best for you, you still have to take daily action to get the best out of your life. This is because family members can be brutally critical of your efforts when the results they get out of your efforts do need meet their emotional and financial needs. Use your self-talk to prepare yourself for the unexpected. Stick to your weight loss goals even if they are not universally approved.

The bottom line is that whether you are dealing with friends, families or co-workers, it is important to make sure you understand the full meaning of your conversations with them. If you are not able to do this you will find yourself constantly having misunderstandings and shouting matches with your friends and loved ones. This will lead to daily anxiety, criticisms and frustrations that can drain your energy and ultimately diminish your ability to lose weight relentlessly unless you change your thought process and make your communication more effective.

If you change your way of thinking, you will change your life and overcome the fear of failure which can stop you from trying your best to lose weight and keep it off. Learn to say "No" to people who are constantly trying to get you to try those snacks you have already told them you do not want because you are trying to lose weight. They may be your friends but they are not helping in your weight-loss journey. They are pointing you in the wrong direction, and listening to them will make you fail.

Picture yourself winning in those scenarios and think deeply about how you would feel after you have successfully lost weight and kept it off. **Celebrate small victories along the way but be prepared for unexpected setbacks.** Having small victories as you pursue your ultimate dream will train you for greater success.

Not everyone will be happy to see that you have not given up on your dreams or that you refuse to let the fear of failure stop you from trying. If you stay focused and refuse to let what others think about you determine how you feel, you will eventually get most of what you want from your daily opportunities.

Don't let your day be full of missed opportunities. Learn to see the possibility for weight loss in every encounter or event that makes up your day. You can do this by directing your energy into making the most out of your daily situations instead of trying to determine whom to blame or whom to chastise. Focus on taking advantage of your daily opportunities rather than on the words and actions of those who generate a lot of negative energy with little or no capacity to support your goals.

Remember that before you can take advantage of your daily opportunities you have to recognize them. You have to know when important opportunities have come your way. Do you look at your daily challenges and setbacks as opportunities to continue with your relentless weight loss program? Do you look at them as proof of your inability to succeed?

If you really want to lose weight relentlessly you have to make consistent adjustments through effective communication strategies. You can do this by making sure that you make your perspectives in such a way that you stay innovative all the time. You cannot allow the fear of failure stop you from trying or prevent you from making full use of your daily opportunities. ***Ozaa Akwusina*** (A warrior never stops).

You have to learn to minimize the tendency to think of the worst outcomes all the time. **Rather than thinking the worst about a situation or an event, remind yourself that remaining positive through difficult times will help you to transform your daily reality. This type of focus will help you to continue to lose weight even if all those around you think that you can't.**

If you do not invest in yourself and in your ability to find out new and better ways to make the most out of your daily opportunities, your dreams and goals will remain illusions to be pursued but ultimately unrealized. You can avoid such an outcome by learning how to spot opportunities and consistently take positive action to transform your opportunities into accomplishments.

You also have to learn how to communicate with yourself and others in a way that makes your relationships mutually beneficial. This will make you feel good about yourself and make you less moody and less likely to eat disruptively. Effective communication strategies are important because according to Burley-Allen (1995), words can affect our biases and lead to uncomfortable emotions and negative reactions. Unfortunately, some of these negative reactions may include giving up on the actions that can help you lose weight because of what others have said or implied. Don't give up. Refocus and evaluate your progress and challenges throughout your weight loss journey!!!

TIPS FOR THE DAY

CELEBRATE WHAT YOU'VE

ACCOMPLISHED AT THE END OF EACH

DAY

DON'T SPEND TOO MUCH TIME LOOKING

BACK,

LOOK FORWARD

TO THE NEXT DAY

Make regular evaluation part of your weight loss strategy

Do you weigh yourself every week? Get a weight-loss journal or notebook. Unless you have a way to regularly evaluate your progress throughout your weight loss journey, you will not have concrete success. How can you tell your daily mini goals if you don't evaluate yourself? Are you regularly eating your variety of vegetables and fruits? Are you still reducing your food portions or have slowly gone back to your old portion? Do you still exercise regularly or have discovered that "you don't have time"? Are you keeping stress out of your relationships and conversations?

To lose weight relentlessly throughout the year you have be able to measure and demonstrate to yourself that what you are doing is working. You have to make your daily mini-goals are subset of your main goal for the week and for the month. If you do not do this, despite your best intentions, you will end up not losing as much weight as you would like to.

After you have determined or discovered the easy activities that will consistently help you to lose weight, take realistic action to transform yourself and get the results you want for yourself. Your goals should be achievable and make sense within the parameters of your life. One way to check your progress in your weight loss journey is to take regular measurements. You can do this by weighing yourself every week, measuring your waist circumference every month and calculating your BMI every six months. You can also use less formal ways like dress size, change in belt hole, pant size, loose ring, or changes in shoe fitting to evaluate your weight loss journey.

Through this book you already know the steps you need to take to help you lose weight every day. Check your list of activities you consider realistic for you to accomplish your weight loss in a day based on your knowledge, experience, personality, available resources and your time –management skills. Once you have a concrete list in front of you, it's a lot easier to check on yourself regularly. You have to stick to your plan and accomplish the tasks on your list one after the other. If you do this day in, day out, week after week, you will easily lose weight throughout the year without gaining it back! Do you have the discipline to do your best with what you have everyday?

TIPS FOR THE DAY

LIMIT INTERRUPTIONS

DON'T BE ON THE PHONE ALL DAY

GET A PLAN AND STICK TO IT

Maintain your discipline and do your best with what you have

Do you remember exactly what you were doing at this time yesterday? Were you losing weight or gaining weight? Did someone make you eat too much or did you resist and eat right? Were you making the best use of your time? Everyone has 24 hours in a day. If you truly want to lose weight, you have to start where you are. Can you find time to walk for five more minutes though your schedule is full? Can you do more to keep stress out of your life? Can you stick to a simple and easy weight loss plan? Are you doing the best with what you have?

The key to making the best out of what you have everyday is discipline. The "O" in the compass method stands for operational capacity profile.

Without a disciplined and focused use of your time and resources your relentless weight loss program will fail. You have to make discipline the anchor of your daily focus. You cannot win without taking consistent action. You cannot achieve your weight loss goals without discipline.

Discipline is like the ladder of success, climbing it one step at a time will help you achieve your goals and much more. If you do not pay attention to your steps as you climb up a ladder, you may end up falling. This means that if you do not have situational awareness while eating, you may eat more than you planned and find yourself gaining weight at the same time. If you truly want to lose weight relentlessly everyday you have to have the situational awareness and discipline to say "No" to friends, coworkers, and well-wishers who want you to try one delightful, amazing delicious food or another!

Without discipline you cannot implement your best ideas for long enough to get the results to help you lose weight and live the lifestyle of your dreams. This means that if you have decided to walk a mile everyday then you have to follow through until you get the benefits you desire. If you have decided to lose weight and keep it off, you have decide on the minimum amount of exercise you shall do everyday and do it. You have to be consistent in keeping your portions small and maintaining the variety of your food with more emphasis on fruits, vegetables and fish.

A disciplined approach to life either through regular exercise or better time management will help you manage stress better and accomplish more throughout the day. This will also help you build up confidence in your ability to carry out your daily weight loss plans. Stress can be very disruptive. It can disrupt your ability to concentrate and stay focused on the task of the moment. It can have an overwhelming and detrimental effect on your lifestyle and confidence. When stress escalates, it throws your whole life out of balance, including your plan to lose weight relentlessly.

This imbalance can occur physically, emotionally and mentally. It can lead to unwanted stress and may even affect your self-confidence and your ability to interact positively with others. This has the potential to lead to negative coping mechanisms like resorting to emotional eating to cope with stress.

When stress leads you to a disruptive place, press the pause button. Trust the process you have already determined works best for you and begin again. Discipline and confidence in yourself will help you determine when to speak, when to listen or when to simply walk away. Constant pressure can occur through your daily interactions and relationships. If you really want to live the lifestyle of your dreams, you have to learn to let things go, and begin to take the daily steps that are productive, constructive and beneficial. Sometimes this simply means giving our loved ones a hug. At other times, it would mean speaking the truth in love or keeping quiet and listening to what others have to say. At other times it may mean walking away from the encounter.

Sometimes this may mean disappointing your friends and your family. It may mean that you cannot attend as many social events as you would like to. It may even mean saying "No" to yourself. Can you do it? Can you withstand the pressure when the negative comments start trickling in? Can you refuse to participate in the activities you really like so that you can focus on the activities that will help you grow? Can you refuse to eat "good" food that may not be good for your own health when everyone around you is asking you to do so? Will you have the discipline to refuse your favorite TV shows or Netflix movie because you watching screen time can lead to unintended consequences? Do you have the discipline to refuse to be distracted by the latest trend or latest "great idea"? When you get to the point where you can more consistently focus and achieve your daily mini-goals you will begin to develop the confidence that will help you to lose weight even when others expect you to fail.

Remember that until you develop enough trust in the way you consistently lose weight that what others say or think won't matter, you won't have enough confidence to lose weight relentlessly throughout the year! The confidence that comes from successful repeated executions of small daily tasks is what will help you put enough trust and confidence in yourself to eliminate unnecessary doubt. Unnecessary doubt is an attribute that will make you double check and triple check your work until you end up making avoidable mistakes, rejecting good products, missing your mini-goals or losing confidence in yourself.

If you lack confidence in yourself and you spend your time and your life seeking approval from others before you complete your projects or try to fulfill your daily dreams and goals, you will be disappointed. You will not be able to relentlessly lose weight because you will unwisely spend most of your time and energy focusing on those who are either not prepared to give you the support you need or frankly lack the ability to give you that support.

Consistent confidence will help you to maintain the discipline that you will need to handle the different circumstances that you will encounter daily life as you remain focused on relentless weight loss. This will help you to overcome the natural tendency to lose confidence when things are not working as you would like them to. It will also help you to pay less emphasis on the results of your efforts and more on the process. **Ask yourself, right now, "Are you making the best possible use of this moment in time?"**

Do not spend your time looking for the perfect plan or start one plan and give it up and start another one? Instead of trying to get the perfect plan or looking for perfect co-workers or perfect friends, do the best you can where you are, with what you have. I know this is a mouthful!! Essentially it boils down to focusing on doing your best with what you have instead of complaining about what you do not have that you could have used to do a better job. You can do this by creating an individualized plan and a mental picture that will help you to maintain a sharp focus on your main goals by breaking them into mini-goals that you can accomplish through small but consistent daily action.

This is actually the key to your ability to relentless weight loss. You have to have the ability to consistently take action that will help you fulfill your goals everyday. If you are not able to do this consistently you will slowly lose confidence in yourself and lack the trust in yourself to do what you have to do to lose weight throughout the year! Can you stay focused and refuse to quit as you continue on your weight loss journey?

TIPS FOR THE DAY

TAKE ONE STEP AT A TIME

PLAN AND ACCOMPLISH YOUR DAILY TASKS

USE CONSISTENT DISCIPLINE TO TRY TO FINISH THE THINGS THAT YOU NEED TO GET DONE

Stay focused and refuse to quit

Do you know that intention is not enough? Can you stay focused on what you had in mind when you started your weight loss journey and refuse to quit? Relentless weight loss throughout the year does not mean that you will not have any failures or disappointments throughout the day. If you want to focus and thrive everyday you have to have a strategic approach to daily living. Here are some strategies that will help you avoid those pitfalls that will make you fail to fulfill your daily goals.

First, focus on the positive and try to be productive everyday because negative thoughts lead to negative emotions and negative outcomes. Lack of focus on the positive leads to poor management of disruptive circumstances and situations. This can to lead to frustrations, anger and less success with weight loss, unless you make adjustments. You have to remember to stay focused and refuse to quit when the going gets tough. Only relentless focus can help accomplish relentless weight loss.

Focus on a step by step approach. First embrace the concept of holistic weight loss through a deeper understanding of your compass profile, then do your 72-hour food audit. Next use the compass "VAM, method to manage your daily meals. After you have gained a more realistic picture of how well you can manage your daily meals, this usually takes about a week or two, set realistic goals for your relentless weight loss program. Do not try to accomplish too many things in a day or you will end up getting yourself overwhelmed and disappointed with little or no time for other parts or aspects of your life.

Do not get into the habit of having too many projects up in the air at once. Finish one before you start another. Begin with end in mind also means that you have a plan for completing your projects when you start them. Don't start your projects with only the hope that you will complete them. Stay focused from the beginning to the end. Write down the day you expect to lose your first 10 pounds after you start. An open –ended weight loss program, discourages completion while promoting lack of focus and delays. If you truly want to transform your life and live the lifestyle of your dreams, you have to be able begin with the end in mind and stay focused on completing your projects or accomplishing your goals one step at a time.

If you truly want to consistently lose weight everyday, you have to refuse to quit after you begin. Too many people begin, then quit before they get the results they desire. You have to be able to strategically put aside your daily disappointments and early failures in your attempts at losing weight. Do not let your daily struggles stop you from focusing on your specific tasks for the day. Be prepared to try your best after the disappointment of the moment or of the hour or of the day. Do you bounce back from adversity everyday? Do you refuse to quit?

Keep in mind that difficult conditions are temporary. **Criticisms will pass if you do not keep replaying them in your mind.** Frustrations will boil over. Focus on your destinations instead of the bumps or delays along your weight loss journey.. **Life is full of ups and downs. Refuse to let a rough morning spoil the rest of your day**. Don't overeat simply because no one seems to appreciate all the effort you have put into losing weight and making yourself morehealthy. When things look bleak, you have to remember that you could be on the verge of a breakthrough. **Never** forget that the darkest part of the night is just before dawn.

Do you take care of your weight? **Do you have a daily plan for dealing with stress?** Do you eat a balanced diet, exercise regularly, and go to bed on time. Do you build the physical and mental strength to keep going when the going gets tough? **Do you bounce refuse to quit when the going gets tough. Do you stay focused?**

If you want to stay focused and refuse to quit everyday, you have to learn to stop being too harsh on yourself and learn to love yourself more everyday. Remember not to allow yourself to be distracted by trying to complete too many projects all at once. Finish one project before you start another. Learn from your mistake. Remember that the relentless weight loss program is a multifaceted process. You have to persist to win.

One of the main reasons why people fail to bounce back everyday is that they are too harsh on themselves. Instead of seeing their short comings as part of the process of growth, they consider them as a confirmation that they can never be successful. You can lose as much weight as you want if you refuse to give up and continue to strive to improve. You can lose weight relentlessly if you follow your own SEPP (Strategy, Effort, Process and Persistence and TIAs (Transformational Infinite Adjustments) that will help you convert obstacles and challenges in your weight loss journey into opportunities for outstanding success. If you do this consistently every week **you will lose weight relentlessly throughout the year!!!**

TIPS FOR THE DAY

UNLESS YOU'RE LOOKING FORWARD TO THE FUTURE, YOU'RE MISERABLE IN THE PRESENT

FOCUS AND PERSIST WITHOUT STOPPING FOR RELENTLESS WEIGHT LOSS

Review and improve (RAI)

Congratulations !!! I am proud of you, for your grit and determination! **After reading this book you have to take action.** First do a one-page review in which you write down everything you have read in this book and how you will use them to lose weight throughout the year.

What is the essence of your holistic weight loss approach? Make this your first paragraph. If you need additional help doing this, visit www.compasswellnessinstitute.com and sign up for my newsletter or simply text me, introducing yourself and asking questions.

Make a list of the barriers to your weight loss program and how you plan to overcome them everyday. If you can't and need more help, please contact me for more *relentless transformational* strategies!

What is your 3-month weight loss goal? Through *relentless loss*, you can lose 10-20 pounds in about 3 months.

What is your biggest challenge or area of frustration?

Slow down so that you can go faster.

Do you like the way you manage stress, time and productivity?

Don't let the perfect become the enemy of the possible.

Persist until success happens (PUSH).

Don't become so afraid of failing that you never begin.

How   can   you   improve?

What changes do you think you can make that will make to relentless weight loss work better for you?

Share your thoughts and concerns by joining the compass club on Facebook so that you find out how others have tackled similar problems or challenges in their weight loss journey.

If you need one on one consultation please visit www.compasswellnessinstitute.com to sign up for the six month relentless weight loss program.

Appendix

Compass Club:I1 week-Motivation Group for Weight loss

Week 1, Education and Measurements.

Through this motivation group participants will remind themselves of why weight loss is a goal for them. Each group member will have a hands on experience of how measurements like waist circumference and body mass index can used to identify whether an individual is within normal weight, overweight, or obese. For this motivation group program the definition of overweight will be based on normal (BMI<25kg/m²), overweight (BMI=25-29 kg/m²), and obesity will be based on a BMI of ≥30. This was the same definition used by Koebnick et al. (2012) in their study on young adults in California. Abdominal obesity will be measured through waist circumference (WC).

Severe abdominal obesity will be defined as (WC $\geq$ 88cm) in women and (WC $\geq$ 102cm) in men.

Week 2, Benefits

Each group member will write down in his weight loss journal the benefits of losing weight, which would include the reduced risk of diabetes, high blood pressure, and heart disease. Those who participate in the program will become more active and spend less time watching television. This will lead to having more time for getting work or studies done. Sleeping more hours per day and eating more healthy food would also reduce the risk of health related problems. Each group member should get their weight loss journal and write down how many hours of sleep, they have every day.

Week 3, Barriers to change

Group members need to remember that the cause of obesity differs for each individual. If it is due to poor eating habits or due to poor physical activity, then it will be easier to change through eating healthy and becoming more active. However, when the cause of obesity or weight gain, includes medical illness like endocrine or neurological problems it becomes more difficult to achieve the desired change. This will require referral to the appropriate health care professional for adequate intervention.

According to Anshel (2010) sometimes the barrier to change is non-adherence to healthy habits. This is one barrier to change that can be modified by self-motivation and working with group members. Encourage one another during your weekly meetings and consider doing healthy competition on weight loss. Make sure there are multiple winners in your group.

Categories can be First to lose 10 pounds

Best fruit salad

Tastiest Lunch

Least expensive fish meal

Most consistent group attendant

Easiest exercise ideas

Best jokes to deal with stress

Your group should aim to award prizes every week, for the first 11-week session of the group.

Week 4 to Week 5

Discuss a selected factor that can influence weight gain as identified through the research. Ask each group member to share their own insight based on what they read about weight loss. Participants will be asked how many hours a day they spent watching television and how much they alcohol and soft drinks they drink weekly.in details per week with given goals. The goal in Week 4 will be focused on cutting down on television time to less than an hour per day, week 5 will be focused on cutting down on the drinking of alcohol and soft drinks to less than 5 times per week.

Week 6: sleep

Week 6 will be focused on increasing sleep to more than 6 hours per day. This will include discussing the role of environmental factors like extended periods of light in the room or changes in room temperature can lead to reduced hours of sleep per day (Knutson,2012). Cultural factors that can influence sleep include how much value the culture or society in which one lives places on health when compared to productivity. If sleep is considered an act of laziness then most people would opt for more work hours and sleep less. Sociocultural conversations on what is normal sleep could also lead to unrealistic expectations and what constitutes normal sleep (Knutson,

2012). This could lead to anxiety and make falling asleep more difficult. Participants will be asked how many hours of sleep they have had each day and what they considered their barriers to sleeping better.

Week 7: diet moderation

Week 7 will be focused on cutting down on sweetened sugars. This is because a study by Bermudez and Gao (2010) found that a greater intake of sweetened beverages was associated with a higher risk of total and abdominal obesity for young adults aged between 20-39 years of age. The study found that 10 additional teaspoons of added sugars per day were associated with a 52% higher risk of obesity. Participants will be asked how teaspoons of added sugar they consumed every day. Their goal would be to reduce the amount of added sugar they consumed every day to less than five teaspoons.

Week 8: Overcoming barriers

Week 8 will focus on increased barriers to physical activity including heightened body consciousness and a feeling of insecurity among those overweight compared to those who were not. It would also be important to allow group members to discuss the role each person's ethnic background has played on how each person feels about his or her weight. This in parts of the world like the pacific Islands find being overweight is more socially acceptable and group members from such places may be less inclined to make too much effort to change or reduce their weight (Stankov, Olds, &Cargo. 2012). Participants will be asked to discuss their feelings about their weight with others and will be encouraged to increase their physical activity by walking at least 30 minutes per day. Participants will also be encouraged to discuss the influence of peer stigmatization in their lives, since research has shown that it is another factor that can prevent participation in regular physical activity

.

Week 9

Week 9 will focus on depressive symptoms. According to Skinner, Haines, Austin, and Field (2011) those complaining of depressive symptoms at baseline were more likely to start overeating. The prevalence of overeating increased from 2.4 % to 3.7% and the percentage of binge eating increased from 2.4% to 5.7%. The prevalence of overweight increased from 14.5% to 15.5% and obesity increased from 3% to 5.2%. Participants will be asked if they have had depressive symptoms in the past and how much they think it has affected them.

Week 10, Focus on Support

Week 10 will focus on support services. Two speakers would be invited to speak to the Participants or two participants will volunteer and do it. These two speakers will focus on helping the participants determine which of the factors discussed in sessions 4 to 9 they feel is most relevant to them and share with them some of the ways they can persevere when they feel like giving up. This is important because according to Anshel (2010), 60 to 70% of adults who begin an exercise program quit in less than a year. A former group participant or someone else who has lost at least 10 pounds and kept it off for at least one year through the compass method can come and share his or her challenges, tribulations and triumphs with the group.

This type of activity prepares the way for both a short term change and a long term change. It is important to remember that obesity frequently becomes a lifelong problem. This is why everyone has to be prepared for a long term process. This will include joining support groups and making changes that fit into a family's lifestyle. Friends of those trying to lose weight can help them improve their self-esteem by emphasizing their strengths and positive qualities rather than just focusing on their weight problems. The more books you read on weight loss, stress management and on personal motivation the more likely you will succeed in your own relentless weight loss program.

Week 11, Review

Week 11 will be a review of what has been done so far. Each participant will be given 5 minutes to share with the group what the 11-week motivation program has meant to him or her. Each participant will also be asked to say what changes they have seen in their lives as a result of their participation in the program. Participants would also be asked to say what challenges remain and what changes they will like to see in the program. Each participant will be weighed and their waist circumference measured, so that their BMI and WC can be compared to what it was at the beginning of

the program. Each participant will be given a certificate of participation and be encouraged to set monthly goals throughout the year. You can also join the compass club on

https://www.facebook.com/groups/174827683543
1116/

for more encouragement and fun activities to help you lose weight and achieve more of your relentless transformation goals and projects.

Notes

American Heart Association (AHA).

American Academy of Child & Adolescence Psychiatry. (2011, March).*Facts for families* (Report No.79). retrieved from http:// www.aacap.org/cs/root/facts_for_families/obesity_in_children.

Anshel, M. H. (2010). The disconnected values (intervention) model for promoting healthy
habits in religious institutions. *Journal of Religion and Health, 49*(1), 32-49.

Burley-Allen, M. (1995). Listening the forgotten skill: a self-teaching guide. New York, NY: John Wiley & Sons, Inc

Center for Disease Control and Prevention (CDC),2017

Pender, N. J., Murdaugh, C.L., & Parsons, M. A. (2011).Health promotion in nursing practice ractice.Boston:Pearson

Samaranayake, N. R., Ong, K. L., Raymond, Y.H. L.,& Chueng, B. M.Y., (2012,May). Management of obesity in the national health and nutrition examination survey (NHANES), 2007–2008. *Annals of Epidemiology, 22*(5),349-353.

Skinner, H.H. , Haines, J., Austin, S. B. , Field, A. E. (2012, May). A prospective study of overeating, binge eating, and depressive symptoms among adolescent and young adult women. *Journal of Adolescent Health, 50* (5), 478–483

Stankov, I., Olds, T., & Cargo, M. (2012). Overweight and obese adolescents: what turns them off physical activity? *The International Journal of Behavioral Nutrition and Physical Activity*, 9 (1)53. Retrieved from http://www.sciencedirect.com.eaproxy.liberty.edu:2048/science/article/pii/0753332294901031

World Health Organization (WHO), 2017

Resources

Get a copy of the weight loss journal and write a letter to yourself on how you plan to stay focused and relentlessly lose weight everyday and throughout year! *Use relentless transformation to Become Unstoppable, Live UnLimited!*

Here are additional resources that will help you to focus and thrive so that you can become the best and happiest version of yourself.

www.compasswellnessinstitute.com

www.compasshealthtransformer.com/members

www.dcompassmarketing.com

http://www.amazon.com/Dr.-Chio-Ugochukwu/e/B00JNFLPQQ

Join the compass club on Facebook

https://www.facebook.com/groups/1748276835431116/

Other books by Dr. Chio Ugochukwu that will help you improve your health, eliminate stress and transform your life include;

The Compass Health Transformer: Your 72 Hour Blue Print For Healthy Living

In this book you will learn more about how doing the 72-hour food audit can help you gain a better understanding of how you can improve your health through easy daily adjustments …..

21 Ways To Transform Your Health Without Medications

"…21 simple proven ways to reduce stress and improve your health and wellbeing without relying on medications. These are easy and effective ways you can use to turn your daily challenges into transformative opportunities for healthy living and daily happiness. You can start right away without spending a fortune!.."

Get your own copy of 21 Ways To Transform Your Health Without Medications

Overcoming Daily Stress: 21 Quick And Easy Ways To Stay Stress-Free In Your Daily Life

"…Are you tired of being stressed out everyday? Are you tired of feeling exhausted and overwhelmed in your daily activities? Are you fed up with communication issues in your relationship? Here are 21 quick and easy ways you can use to overcome daily stress and turn your daily challenges into opportunities for transformative abundant living. This book will help you gain a better understanding of your potential communication issues, daily 'stress points' and the steps you can take to overcome them…".

Get your own copy of Overcoming Daily Stress

The Secret To Daily happiness

"..Have you ever wondered why daily happiness has continued to elude you? Do you want to make sustainable daily happiness part of your life? By reading this book you can find answers to these questions and many more on how to overcome the many obstacles and challenges that daily try to take away your inner peace and contentment…"

Get your own copy of The Secret To Happiness

15 Simple Ways to lower your blood pressure naturally after 40 without complicated diets

"……Don't spend your most productive years dealing with high blood pressure, medications and side effects. Stop worrying about whether you forgot to take your first medication or the second one. Take these simple steps to lower your blood pressure naturally and minimize your need for multiple medications. Did you know that high blood pressure can cause heart attack, stroke, kidney failure, blindness and memory problems? Don't wait to find out! Take Action! ,,,,,"

Click Here for Your own copy of 15 Simple Ways To Reduce Blood Pressure....

Here is a book to help lose fat. If your main concern or focus is losing pounds you have accumulated as fat then get a copy of the book

"How To Lose 23 Pounds of Fat Without Torture Diets or Hard Exercise And keep it (The Compass Method).

"Are you fed up with trying to lose weight again and again with limited success? Are you tired of all the confusing new and expensive diets you have tried to follow every day with zero results? Do you want the health benefits of living with optimum weight without following complicated rules? Do you want to become more energetic and active again? Are you fed up with the wild ride of losing weight today and gaining it back tomorrow? Then read this book so that you will start using a comprehensive individualized weight loss strategy that will help you lose fat and keep it off, without going on torture diets or deadly strenuous exercises. You will learn to do this through the Compass Method that is based on a holistic approach to weight-loss, healthy living and personal transformation."

If prayer is something that appeals to you, you might be interested in the following next two books that incorporate prayers into our daily strive to become better and become more fulfilled:

Praying To Win: How To Get More Victories And Riches In Your Daily Life Through Spiritual Principles

"..You too can achieve your goals and dreams, through praying to win. You can do this by immersing yourself in the word of God and transforming the moments that make up your daily life through persistent adoration……. Above all, thank God every day, never give up and persistently continue praying to win…"

Get your own copy of Praying To Win

9 Best Ways To Eliminate Stress, Improve Your Health And thrive Without Limitations Through Prayers

Are tired of being knocked down by stress from your daily hassles? Are you tired of dealing with chronic illnesses associated with stress? Do you want to live a fun-filled daily life? Here are 9 of the best ways you can change your daily obstacles and challenges into opportunities to thrive without limitations through the power of prayers.

Too Young To Die

"A book about coping with grief and finding your way in life…"

9 Best Ways To Quit Smoking Without Becoming A Nervous Wreck And Gaining Weight

"..Here are 9 of the best ways to finally quit smoking without becoming a nervous wreck or gaining weight. If you have tried to quit smoking before, but failed or tried to quit but was overcome by anxiety or fear of becoming socially awkward or gaining weight, then read this book! This book was previously published as "The Compass Health Transformer Quit Smoking", but has been rewritten to include the transtheoretical model of change to help you get a better understanding of where you are in your journey or process of quitting smoking. The 9 best ways to quit smoking also includes a reminder of the different ways smoking can affect your health and body and the different individualized-changes you can make to your life-style to help you quit smoking on your own terms.

9 Best Ways To Deal With Negative People, Protect Your Health And Be Happy

"..Are you tired of being stressed out by encounters with negative people? Are you fed up with the impact of negative situations on your health and happiness? Would like you to find out ways to remain effective during negative situations and encounters with negative people? Do you know that chronic stress generated by negative encounters can damage your eyes, heart and brain? Do you know that chronic stress can directly damage your body cells? Here are 9 best ways you can protect your health from such negative situations so that you can continue to thrive and be happy..".

Are You Tough Enough To Be Great?

"..Have you discovered what you really want in life? Have you discovered why you were born? Do you know the direction you are going with your life….Learn more about how you can use the growth mindset to help you strive to excel in everything that you do in spite of distractions and challenges....You will discover more strategies that will help you seek excellence in everything that you do so that **you can become unstoppable and live unlimited! BULU!! Become Unstoppable, Live Unlimited. BULU!!!**

To order new or additional copies or ask questions, please visit:

http://www.amazon.com/Dr.-Chio-Ugochukwu/e/B00JNFLPQQ

Call or Text : 661 992 6436

You can also get courses on wellness and transformational living from

www.compasswellnessinstitute.com/courses

Join the Compass club @

https://www.facebook.com/compassclub

About the Author

Dr. Chio Ugochukwu has always been interested in empowering people to improve their health, keep stress out of their relationships, live the lives they intended, and transform their communication and leadership skills through **relentless transformation**. He has inspired many people to discover their passion and purpose and drive themselves to greater achievement and transformation despite their busy schedules, daily challenges and duties.

He was inspired to develop *The Compass Method for Relentless Transformation*, through his ancient heritage of *Ozaa Akwusina* (Warriors Never Stop) and the challenges he has encountered in his journey of life, his practice of medicine and his fascination with how effective communications, the mind, the spirit and human experience influence the accomplishment of goals and the fulfillment of life. You can find out more about the Compass Method and other courses and programs for **relentless transformation** by Dr. Chio by visiting www.compasswellnessinstitute.com.

As an author and researcher, he has published many books, with peer-reviewed publications on quality of life and numerous articles on stress, communications, healthy living and relentless transformation. He is the medical director of Dala Compass Foundation and a consultant with the Compass Consultants International (CCI). As a consultant and specialist, he is focused on helping individuals and organizations achieve their goals through their own customized strategic pathways for **relentless transformation**.